BRIGHTON'S GUIDE TO

1st Edition

Top 350 Medications with Usual and Renal dosing

Review of Laboratory Tests and Monitoring Parameters

Editor:

Dr. Brighton Abebe, PharmD
and Negussie Abebe

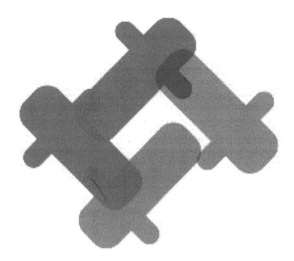

BRIGHTON GUIDE is published by:

Boku Publishing, INC
New York, NY
Email: info@brightonguide.com

Note to Readers
We welcome questions comments and feedback concerning the guide. All of your feedbacks are reviewed and taken into account in updating the content of the guide. This guide has made every effort to insure the accuracy of the information. However, the editors and publishers are not responsible for errors or omissions or for any consequence from application of the information in this book and make no warranty, express or implied, with respect to the accuracy, or completeness of the content of this publication. Application of this information remains the professional responsibility of the practitioner.

ISBN: 9781098749682

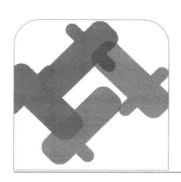

Introduction

Ranking of TOP 300 Drugs for 2019

1	Levothyroxine	55	Norethindrone/Ethinyl Estradiol
2	Lisinopril	56	Ergocalciferol
3	Atorvastatin	57	Lorazepam
4	Metformin Hydrochloride	58	Norgestimate/ Ethinyl Estradiol
5	Amlodipine Besylate	59	Estradiol
6	Metoprolol	60	Triamterene/Hydrochlorothiazide
7	Omeprazole	61	Glimepiride
8	Simvastatin	62	Salmeterol Xinafoate/ Fluticasone
9	Losartan Potassium	63	Diltiazem Hydrochloride
10	Albuterol	64	Paroxetine
11	Gabapentin	65	Loratadine
12	Hydrochlorothiazide	66	Spironolactone
13	Hydrocodone/Acetaminophen	67	Fenofibrate
14	Sertraline Hydrochloride	68	Naproxen
15	Furosemide	69	Esomeprazole
16	Fluticasone	70	Lamotrigine
17	Acetaminophen	71	Metronidazole
18	Amoxicillin	72	Lovastatin
19	Alprazolam	73	Alendronate Sodium
20	Atenolol	74	Cetirizine Hydrochloride
21	Citalopram	75	Finasteride
22	Insulin Glargine	76	Clonidine
23	Montelukast	77	Formoterol/ Budesonide
24	Trazodone Hydrochloride	78	Diclofenac
25	Pantoprazole Sodium	79	Latanoprost
26	Escitalopram Oxalate	80	Losartan Potassium/ Hydrochlorothiazide
27	Pravastatin Sodium	81	Bacitracin/Neomycin/ Polymyxin B
28	Bupropion	82	Sitagliptin Phosphate
29	Fluoxetine Hydrochloride	83	Pregabalin
30	Carvedilol	84	Insulin Humulin
31	Prednisone	85	Topiramate
32	Tamsulosin Hydrochloride	86	Quetiapine Fumarate
33	Potassium	87	Insulin Aspart
34	Clopidogrel Bisulfate	88	Amitriptyline
35	Ibuprofen	89	Levetiracetam
36	Meloxicam	90	Buspirone Hydrochloride
37	Rosuvastatin Calcium	91	Ondansetron
38	Aspirin	92	Valsartan
39	Tramadol Hydrochloride	93	Ferrous Sulfate
40	Zolpidem Tartrate	94	Enalapril Maleate
41	Warfarin	95	Tiotropium
42	Clonazepam	96	Folic Acid
43	Propranolol Hydrochloride	97	Hydroxyzine
44	Glipizide	98	Donepezil Hydrochloride
45	Dextroamphetamine; Amphetamine	99	Lisdexamfetamine Dimesylate
46	Cyclobenzaprine	100	Insulin Lispro
47	Methylphenidate	101	Isosorbide Mononitrate
48	Duloxetine	102	Ciprofloxacin
49	Azithromycin	103	Cholecalciferol
50	Ranitidine	104	Benazepril Hydrochloride
51	Venlafaxine Hydrochloride	105	Rivaroxaban
52	Allopurinol	106	Trimethoprim Sulfamethoxazole
53	Lisinopril/ Hydrochlorothiazide	107	Cephalexin
54	Oxycodone	108	Oxybutynin

Ranking of TOP 300 Drugs for 2019

109	Drospirenone/ Ethinyl Estradiol	163	Levocetirizine Dihydrochloride
110	Doxycycline	164	Olmesartan Medoxomil
111	Ropinirole Hydrochloride	165	Mometasone
112	Diazepam	166	Ipratropium Bromide/ Albuterol
113	Hydrocodone Bitartrate	167	Brimonidine Tartrate
114	Amoxicillin/Clavulanate potassium	168	Valacyclovir
115	Sumatriptan	169	Terazosin
116	Pioglitazone	170	Solifenacin Succinate
117	Levonorgestrel/ Ethinyl Estradiol	171	Irbesartan
118	Tizanidine	172	Glyburide
119	Thyroid	173	Fluconazole
120	Celecoxib	174	Chlorthalidone
121	Insulin Detemir	175	Carbidopa/Levodopa
122	Triamcinolone	176	Beclomethasone
123	Apixaban	177	Polyethylene Glycol 3350
24	Baclofen	178	Dicyclomine Hydrochloride
125	Famotidine	179	Magnesium
126	Nebivolol Hydrochloride	180	Nitroglycerin
127	Docusate	181	Carisoprodol
128	Mirtazapine	182	Ipratropium
129	Divalproex Sodium	183	Cholecalciferol Calcium
130	Verapamil Hydrochloride	184	Clobetasol Propionate
131	Aripiprazole	185	Temazepam
132	Gemfibrozil	186	Nitrofurantoin
133	Desogestrel/Ethinyl Estradiol	187	Methocarbamol
134	Valsartan/Hydrochlorothiazide	188	Liraglutide
135	Hydroxychloroquine Sulfate	189	Progesterone
136	Prednisolone	190	Dexlansoprazole
137	Cyanocobalamin	191	Metformin/Sitagliptin Phosphate
138	Hydralazine Hydrochloride	192	Nortriptyline Hydrochloride
139	Omega-3-acid Ethyl Esters	193	Benzonatate
140	Benazepril/Amlodipine Besylate	194	Canagliflozin
141	Lansoprazole	195	Acyclovir
142	Timolol	196	Linagliptin
143	Hydrocortisone	197	Carbamazepine
144	Ezetimibe	198	Amiodarone Hydrochloride
145	Digoxin	199	Mupirocin
146	Testosterone	200	Timolol Maleate / Dorzolamide
147	Memantine Hydrochloride	201	Phenytoin
148	Methylprednisolone	202	Butalbital/ Acetaminophen
149	Estrogens Conjugated	203	Mometasone Furoate/ Formoterol
150	Adalimumab	204	Pramipexole Dihydrochloride
151	Clindamycin	205	Ketoconazole
152	Methotrexate	206	Naphazoline Hydrochloride/ Pheniramine
153	Ramipril	207	Budesonide
154	Nifedipine	208	Quinapril
155	Methylcellulose	209	Dexmethylphenidate Hydrochloride
156	Guanfacine	210	Diphenhydramine Hydrochloride
157	Doxazosin Mesylate	211	Benztropine Mesylate
158	Morphine	212	Hydromorphone Hydrochloride
159	Risperidone	213	Cyclosporine
160	Promethazine Hydrochloride	214	Etonogestrel/Ethinyl Estradiol
161	Levofloxacin	215	Sodium Fluoride
162	Meclizine Hydrochloride	216	Lidocaine

217	Nystatin	270	Sotalol Hydrochloride
218	Fentanyl	271	Dorzolamide Hydrochloride
219	Azathioprine	272	Desvenlafaxine
220	Prazosin Hydrochloride	273	Flecainide Acetate
221	Sodium	274	Dutasteride
222	Lithium	275	Methimazole
223	Levonorgestrel	276	Ranolazine
224	Anastrozole	277	Niacin
225	Olanzapine	278	Vilazodone Hydrochloride
226	Phentermine	279	Terbinafine
227	Lurasidone Hydrochloride	280	Tadalafil
228	Cefdinir	281	Erythromycin
229	Minocycline Hydrochloride	282	Bisoprolol Fumarate
230	Chlorhexidine	283	Nadolol
231	Calcitriol	284	Modafinil
232	Rizatriptan Benzoate	285	Rabeprazole Sodium
233	Labetalol	286	Eszopiclone
234	Torsemide	287	Sennosides
235	Penicillin V	288	Prochlorperazine
236	Sucralfate	289	Empagliflozin
237	Primidone	290	Neomycin/Polymyxin B/Hydrocortisone
238	Tamoxifen Citrate	291	Cefuroxime
239	Doxepin Hydrochloride	292	Amphetamine
240	Mesalamine	293	Exenatide
241	Codeine Phosphate/ Guaifenesin	294	Raloxifene Hydrochloride
242	Sildenafil acetate	295	Enoxaparin Sodium
243	Haloperidol	296	Ketorolac Tromethamine
244	Oxcarbazepine	297	Tretinoin
245	Atomoxetine Hydrochloride	298	Atropine/ diphenoxylate Hydrochloride
246	Telmisartan	299	Ofloxacin
247	Calcium	300	Tolterodine Tartrate
248	Travoprost		
249	Oseltamivir Phosphate		
250	Metoclopramide Hydrochloride		
251	Colchicine		
252	Medroxyprogesterone Acetate		
253	Epinephrine		
254	Bimatoprost		
255	Pancrelipase Lipase/ Protease/ Amylase		
256	Loperamide Hydrochloride		
257	Liothyronine Sodium		
258	Olmesartan/Hydrochlorothiazide		
259	Dexamethasone 1		
260	Vortioxetine Hydrobromide		
261	Guaifenesin		
262	Chlorthalidone/Atenolol		
263	Mirabegron		
264	Cilostazol		
265	Norethindrone		
266	Bumetanide		
267	Azelastine Hydrochloride		
268	Dabigatran Etexilate Mesylate		
269	Olopatadine		

TOP 301 – 350 are discussed later and have a symbol (***) to indicate their designation

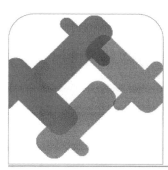

Review Of Laboratory Test

BASIC METABOLIC PANEL (BMP)

	FUNCTION	VALUE	ELEVATED	DECREASED
Sodium (Na)	Extracellular cation	135-145 mEq/L	"Hypernatremia" Fluid loss/ dehydration Diabetes insipidus Hyperaldosteronis	"Hyponatremia" Excess body water CHF
Potassium (K)	Intracellular cation Regulates cardiac, nerve, and muscle function	3.5-5.0 mEq/L	"Hyperkalemia" Acidosis Renal failure	"Hypokalemia" Diarrhea Vomiting Respiratory alkalosis
Chloride (Cl)	Extracellular anion	95-106 mEq/L	"Hyperchloremia" Metabolic acidosis Respiratory alkalosis Renal disorders	"Hypochloremia" Vomiting Metabolic alkalosis
HCO₃		22-30 mEq/L	Metabolic alkalosis	Metabolic acidosis
Blood urea nitrogen (BUN)	Protein catabolism product Produced in the liver Cleared by kidneys	6-20 mg/dL	"Azotemia" Renal failure Dehydration	Liver failure Acromegaly SIADH
Creatinine (SCr)	Muscle breakdown product Marker of renal function	0.6-1.2 mg/dL	Renal dysfunction Dehydration (BUN:SCr >20:1)	Cachexia Immobility
Glucose	Energy source	70-130 mg/dL	"Hyperglycemia" Diabetes mellitus	"Hypoglycemia" Addison disease

OTHER ELECTROLYTES

	FUNCTION	VALUE	ELEVATED	DECREASED
Calcium (Ca)	Found in bones and teeth Corrected calcium = measured Ca + (0.8 x [0.4 – albumin])	**Total calcium: 8.5-10.5 mg/dL** **Free Ca = 1.1-1.4 mmol/L, 4**	"Hypercalcemia" Primary hyperparathyroidism Malignancy Drugs	"Hypocalcemia" Hypoparathyroidism Vitamin D deficiency Hyperphosphatemia Alcoholism Drugs
Magnesium (Mg)	Cofactor for energy utilization Muscle contraction Carbohydrate metabolism Nucleic acid synthesis	**1.7-2.3 mg/dL**	"Hyper-magnesemia" Renal failure Addison's disease Drugs	"Hypomagnesemia" Diarrhea Vomiting Renal wasting Malabsorption Drugs
Phosphate (PO₄)	Intracellular anion Necessary for energy and phospholipid formation	**2.5-5 mg/dL**	"Hyperphosphatemia" Renal dysfunction Increased vitamin D intake Hypoparathyroidism	"Hypophosphatemia" Alcoholism Malnutrition Respiratory alkalosis Hyperparathyroidism

LIVER PANEL

	FUNCTION	VALUE	ELEVATED
Total protein	Protein status	6-8 g/dL 60-80 g/L	Blood cancers Dehydration
Albumin	Protein status Fluid distribution	3.5-5 g/dL	Dehydration
Prealbumin	Nutrition	15-35 mg/dL	
Aspartate amino-transferase (AST)	Found in heart, kidney, pancreas, lungs, muscle	0-40 U/L	Hepatocellular disease Trauma, CHF, MI, Drugs
Alanine amino-transferase (ALT)	Liver metabolism Only in liver	0-55 U/L	Hepatocellular disease Drugs
Alkaline phosphatase (AP)	Dephosphorylation Found in bone, liver, biliary tract	50-130 U/L	Biliary obstruction Bone and Liver disease
Total bilirubin (T$_{bili}$)	Hemoglobin breakdown product	0.1-1 mg/dL	May cause jaundice
Indirect bilirubin	"unconjugated bili"	0.2-0.7 mg/dL	Hemolysis Pernicious anemia
Direct bilirubin (D$_{bili}$)	"conjugated bili"	0-0.2 mg/dL	Hepatocellular disease Cholestasis
Amylase	Digestion of complex carbohydrates	20-130 U/L	Pancreatitis and Cholecystitis
Lipase	Digestion of fats	1.160 U/L	Pancreatitis and Cholecystitis

COMPLETE BLOOD COUNT (CBC)

	FUNCTION	VALUE	ELEVATED	DECREASED
Neutrophils	Bacterial and fungal infections, inflammation	**40-70%** 1.5-7 x10^3 cells/mm^3	Infection Stress response Inflammation Medications	Overwhelming infection Hepatitis Some viral infections Drugs
Lymphocytes	Immune response	**20-40%** 1-5 x10^3 cells/mm^3	Hepatitis, Leukemia Multiple myeloma	Acute infections HIV
Monocytes	Mature into macrophages, Scavenger foreign substances	**2-8%** 0-0.8 x10^3 cells/mm^3	Mycobacterium tuberculosis	
Eosinophils	Phagocytes, kill bacteria and yeast; involved in allergic reactions and immune response to parasites	**0-6%** 0-0.5 x10^3 cells/mm^3	Allergies, asthma Infections and drugs	
Basophils	Phagocytes, associated with hypersensitivity reactions	**<1%** 0-0.2 x10^3 cells/mm^3	Hypersensitivity reactions	
Red Blood Cells (CBC)	Transport Oxygen	4.3 – 5.9 million cells/mm^3 (male) 3.5 – 5.5 million cells/mm^3 (Female)	Polycythemia vera High altitude Strenuous exercise	Anemia Lymphoma Leukemia
Hemoglobin (Hgb)	Oxygen-carrying component of RBCs	14-18 g/dL (male) 12-16 g/dL (female)	COPD, Smokers, High altitude Polycythemia vera	Anemia, Blood loss Hemolysis, Pregnancy, fluid
Hematocrit (Hct)	Vol. of blood occupied by RBCs	39-50 % (male) 33-45 % (female)	COPD, Smokers, High altitude Polycythemia vera	Anemia, Blood loss, Cirrhosis, Hyperthyroid, Leukemia, Pregnancy
Platelets (Plt)	For blood clot formation	150-450 x 10^3 cells/mL	Malignancy, Chronic Inflammation	Cirrhosis, Heparin Induced Thrombocytopenia (HIT), CHEMO

PATHOLOGICAL LABORATORY APPROACH

DISORDER	COMMON LABS	IMPORTANCE
Cardio	Troponin, creatinine kinase (CK), creatinine kinase-muscle and brain (CKMB)	Evaluation for acute coronary syndromes; checked in setting of chest pain
	Lipid panel Total cholesterol [TC], low density lipoprotein [LDL], high density lipoprotein [HDL], triglycerides	Evaluation of cardiovascular risk TG: also elevated in pancreatitis
Hematologic	Iron panel ferritin, total iron binding capacity [TIBC], iron (Fe)	Diagnosis of anemias, hemochromatosis, cancers
	Vitamin B12	Diagnosis of anemia, B12 deficiency
	Prothrombin time (PT), International normalized ratio (INR) Activated partial thromboplastin time (aPTT)	Evaluation of anticoagulation with various drugs, bleeding risk
Endocrine	Hemoglobin A1c	Diagnosis of diabetes mellitus
	Cortisol	Adrenal gland disorders such as Cushing disease, Addison disease
	Thyroid stimulating hormone (TSH) Free T_4	Low indicates hypothyroidism High indicates hyperthyroidism
GI	Stool guaiac AKA fecal occult blood test (FOBT) AKA hemoccult test	Detects blood in the stool indicating GI bleed
MS	T-score	Osteoporosis
Neuro	Lumbar puncture, "spinal tap"	Detects infection, electrolyte abnormalities
Urinary	Urinalysis	Detects infection (WBCs, bacteria), kidney disease (albumin, protein), hyperglycemic crises (ketones, glucose)

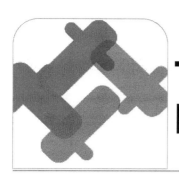

TABLE 1: CARDIAC
Medications

TABLE 1.1: ANTIANGINALS, ANTIARRYTHMICS HEMATOLOGICAL

Medication Name		DRUG CLASS	ADVERSE REACTION
generic	BRAND®		
isosorbide mononitrate	IMDUR	Vasodilator (veins)	Headache Dizziness
nitroglycerin SL, SPRY, Packets	NITROSTAT NITROQUICK	Vasodilator Anti-ischemia	Headache, Dizziness Flushing
ranolazine	RANEXA	Vasodilator Anti-ischemia	Bradycardia Hypotension
amiodarone	PACERONE CORDARONE	Class III	Hypotension, Heart Failure Cardiogenic shock/arrest
digoxin Tab, Inj	LANOXIN		Bradycardia, Blurry vision
opafenone	RYTHMOL	Class IC	Dizziness Taste disturbances
sotalol	BETAPACE	Class II & III	Pro-arrhythmia, Torsade De Pointes
clopidogrel	PLAVIX	Antiplatelet	Bleeding, hematoma, pruritus
aspirin		Antiplatelet	Bleeding, Dyspepsia, **Take with Food**
apixaban	ELIQUIS	Factor Xa inhibitor	
rivaroxaban	XARELTO	Factor Xa inhibitor	Bleeding, Hematoma, **Monitor: CBC** and **Renal**
dabigatran CAP	PRADAXA	Direct thrombin	Bleeding, Hematoma, Dyspepsia
warfarin	Coumadin	Vitamin K Epoxide Reductase inhib.	Bleeding, Skin necrosis Purple toe syndrome (rare)
**dipyridamole and aspirin	AGGRENOX	Antiplatelets	Bleeding, Dyspepsia, **Take with Food**

TABLE 1.2: ANTIHYPERTENSIVES

Medication Name		DOSING	ADVERSE REACTION (AE)
generic	**BRAND®**		
ANGIOTENSIN I INHIBITORS (ACEi)			
Block the conversion of **angiotensin I to angiotensin II**, leading to an increase in blood flow by decreasing vasoconstriction and aldosterone secretion.			
benazepril	LOTENSIN	5-40 mg daily (QD) **CrCl <50: 5 mg**	**AE:** Cough (persistent and dry) Hyperkalemia, Headache Angioedema (<2% rare) Neutropenia, Agranulocytosis, Proteinuria Glomerulonephritis, Acute Kidney Disease (AKI)
donepezil	ARICEPT	5-10 mg daily **CrCl <50: 5 mg**	
enalapril Tablet, Oral	VASOTEC, EPANED	5-20 mg QD **CrCl<10: 2.5-5 mg**	
**fosinopril	MONOPRIL	10-40 mg daily No renal issue	**Boxed:** can cause fetus injury when used in 2nd and 3rd trimesters.
lisinopril Tablet, Oral	ZESTRIL, PRINIVIL, QBRELIS	5-40 mg daily **CrCl <50: 5 mg**	**Contraindications (CI)** Bilateral renal artery stenosis History of angioedema **Avoid in pregnancy**
quinapril	ACCUPRIL	5-40 mg daily **CrCl < 10: 5 mg**	**Monitoring:** BP, Electrolytes (K+) LFTs (Liver) SCr, BUN (renal)
ramipril	ALTACE	5-20 mg QD **CrCL <50: 5 mg**	
ANGIOTENSIN II RECEPTOR BLOCKER (ARBs)			
As a selective and competitive, nonpeptide angiotensin II receptor antagonist, blocks the vasoconstrictor and aldosterone-secreting effects of angiotensin II; interacts reversibly at the AT1 and AT2 receptors of many tissues and has slow dissociation kinetics; its affinity for the AT1 receptor is 1000 times greater than the AT2 receptor.			
irbesartan	AVAPRO	75-300 daily	**AE:** Hyperkalemia, Angioedema (cross-reactivity has been reported) Dizziness, Headache
losartan	COZAAR	25-100 mg daily	
olmesartan	BENICAR	10-40 mg daily	**Boxed:** can cause fetus injury when used in 2nd and 3rd trimesters. **Monitoring:** BP, K+ and SCr & BUN (renal fxn)
valsartan	DIOVAN	80-320 mg daily	

TABLE 1.3: ANTIHYPERTENSIVES

Medication Name		DOSING	ADVERSE REACTION (AE)
generic	BRAND®		
Beta blockers end in "-lol" and inhibit the beta receptor on smooth muscle and myocardial cells; this causes vasodilation.			
NON-SELECTIVE BETA AND ALPHA-1 BLOCKER			
carvedilol Tablet, ER, CAPs	COREG COREG CR	6.25-25 mg BID 20 – 80 mg daily	Edema Weight gain, Increase Triglycerides, Decrease HDL
labetalol Tablet, Inj	NORMODYNE TRANDATE	100-1,200 mg BID	**CI:** hepatic impairment **Take with Food**
BETA-1 CARDIO SELECTIVE BLOCKERS			
atenolol	TENORMIN	5-100 mg QD or BID or TID **CrCl <50: 2.5-50 mg**	Bradycardia Hypotension, Fatigue Dizziness, depression
bisoprolol	ZEBETA ZIAC	2.5-10 mg daily **CrCl <50: 5 mg**	Decreased libido impotence
metoprolol succinate	TOPROL XL Tablet	25-400 mg daily CHF: 12.5-200 mg QD	**Boxed**: Do not discontinue abruptly, taper over 1-2weeks
metoprolol tartrate	LOPRESSOR Tablet, INJ	100-450 mg daily BID or TID	**Take with Food**
nebivolol	BYSTOLIC	5-40 mg daily	
NON-SELECTIVE BETA-1 AND BETA-2 BLOCKERS			
propranolol Tablet, ER, Cap, Oral, Inj.	INDERAL LA INDERAL XL INNOPRAN XL	80-640 mg daily BID 80-120 mg daily	same as above plus Hyperglycemia in diabetics Cross BBB
	Caution: in asthma and severe COPD due to pulmonary beta-blockage. Beta Blockers enhance the hypoglycemic effect of insulin and sulfonylureas and can mask symptoms of **hypoglycemia (shakiness, palpitations, anxiety)** but does not mask **sweating or hunger** More orthostatic hypotension with mixed α and β-blockers. To avoid rebound HTN, dose tapered gradually over 1-2 weeks. For patient with CHF only **bisoprolol**, **carvedilol** and **metoprolol succinate** are recommended. **Monitoring: BP, HR, SCr, BUN**		
DIHYDROPYRIDINES CALCIUM CHANNEL BLOCKERS (CCB)			
DHP CCBs end in "-pine" and inhibit Ca+ ions from entering vascular smooth muscle and myocardial cells; this causes peripheral arterial vasodilation.			
amlodipine	NORVASC	5-10 mg daily	**AE:** Peripheral edema, Dizziness, Flushing, Headache, Palpitations, Gingival Hyperplasia
nifedipne	PROCARDIA (XL) ADALAT CC	30-90 mg daily	**Monitoring:** BP, HR, peripheral edema (lower legs)

TABLE 1.4: ANTIHYPERTENSIVES

Medication Name		DOSING	ADVERSE REACTION
generic	**BRAND®**		
NON-DIHYDROPYRIDINES CALCIUM CHANNEL BLOCKERS (non-DHP CCB)			
diltiazem Tablet, Caps, Inj	CARDIZEM-24H	120-360 mg daily	**AE:** Bradycardia, AV block, Anorexia, Nausea, ****Gingival Hyperplasia more common with non DHP CCB
verapamil Tablet, Caps, Inj	CALAN, COVERA HS	240-480 mg QHS	**Contraindications:** Afib/flutter, CHF (HFrEF), cardiogenic shock; 2nd or 3rd degree AV block. **Monitoring:** HR, Edema, BP, ECG, LFTs
DIURETICS			
Inhibits Na^+/Cl^- reabsorption in the ascending loop of Henle and proximal renal tubule.			
bumetanide	BUMEX No adjustment	0.2-10mg BID No renal adjustment	**AE:** Volume depletion Electrolyte imbalance
furosemide	LASIX	20-80mg daily or BID No renal adjustment	Dizziness, Ringing in the ears Less hyperglycemia
metolazone	ZAROXOLYN	2.5 – 5 mg daily Avoid CrCl < 30 ml/min	Chest pain, chills, depression, pruritus
	Monitoring: BP, electrolytes, BUN, SCr, LFTs, fluid status (Ins/Outs, weight), ototoxicity		
THIAZIDE DIURETICS			
Excretion of salt (Na^+ Cl^-), water, K^+ and H^+ ions at the distal convoluted tubules. Has chronic antihypertensive effects due to an increase in			
hydrochloro-thiazide Tablet, Caps	MICROZIDE ESIDRIX	12.5-25 mg daily **CrCl<30:** **Not effective**	**Sulfa allergy**, photosensitivity Hypokalemia, Hyponatremia, Hypomagnesemia, Hypercalcemia, Hyperuricemia Elevated LDL, TG, BG
chlorthalidone	HYGROTON		
	Monitoring: BP, electrolytes, BUN, SCr, fluid status (Ins/Outs, weight) BG (in diabetics)		
POTASSIUM SPARING			
Competes with aldosterone for receptor sites in the distal renal tubules, increasing salt (Na, Cl) and water while conserving K and H ions.			
spironolactone	ALDACTONE	50-100mg QD or BID **CrCl 10-50: q12-24h** **CrCL <10: avoid**	Fatigue, Hyperkalemia, Glynecomastia **Contraindications**: Anuria, Hyperkalemia, K+ supplements

TABLE 1.6: ANTIHYPERTENSIVES

Medication Name			
generic	BRAND®	DOSING/Class	ADVERSE REACTION
COMBINATION ANTIHYPERTENSIVES			
atenolol/chlorthalidone	TENORETIC	BB + HCTZ	**AE:** Bradycardia, Hypotension, Fatigue
amlodipine/benzepril	LOTREL	CCB + ACEi	Edema, Cough, Flushing
losartan/HCTZ	HYZAAR	ARBs + HCTZ	Hyperkalemia, Angioedema, Dizziness, Headache
olmesartan/HCTZ	BENICAR HCT	ARBs + HCTZ	
valsartan/HCTZ	DIOVAN HCT	ARBs + HCTZ	
lisinopril/HCTZ	ZESTORETIC	ACEi + HCTZ	
triamterene/HCTZ	DYAZIDE	DIURETICS	**Sulfa allergy**, Hypokalemia
ALPHA (α) 1 ANTAGONIST BLOCKERS			
Peripheral inhibition of norepinephrine uptake at α-1 receptors in smooth muscle cells; resulting in vasodilation and lowering blood pressure. **NOTE:** can also be used in men with BPH; relaxes smooth muscle in bladder neck and prostate by inhibiting post-synaptic α- receptors			
doxazosin	CARDURA CARDURA (XL)	IR: 1-16 mg QD XL: 4-8 mg QD	Orthostatic hypotension First dose syncope Cross the BBB (vivid dreams)
prazosin	MINIPRESS	1-20 mg BID, TID	Priapism (prolonged erection) **Contraindication:** Doxazosin with strong **3A4** inhibitors
terazosin	HYTRIN	1-20 mg QHS, BID	
CENTRALLY ACTING ALPHA (α) 2 AGONIST			
Direct stimulation of α2 adrenergic receptors in the vasomotor center of the medulla of the brain to reduces sympathetic outflow. Thus, reduction in peripheral vascular resistance leads to decrease in blood pressure.			
clonidine Tablet patch Inj.	CATAPRES NEXICLON XR -TTS patch	0.1– 2.4 BID 0.17-0.52 mg QD 0.1-0.3 mg /24Hr/Wk	Anticholinergic effects (Dry mouth, Drowsiness, Constipation) Dry eyes, Fatigue, Hypotension, depression **Patch:** Skin (Pruritus, Erythema)
DIRECT VASODILATORS			
Direct vasodilation of arterioles with little effect on veins, causing a decrease in SVR, and blood pressure.			
hydralazine Tablet, Inj.	APRESOLINE	PO 10-300 mg BID IV 10-20mg Q4-6H PRN	Headache, Hypotension, Palpitations, Peripheral neuritis Drug-induced lupus (dose) **Boxed:** pericardial effusion
	Contraindications: CAD, Rheumatic Fever. **Monitoring:** CBC, BP		

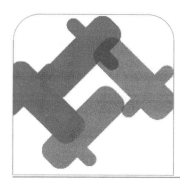# Table 2: Endocrine and Hormonal Agents

TABLE 2.1: ANTIDIABETICS

Medication Name		DOSING	ADVERSE REACTION
generic	BRAND®		
BIGUANIDES (A1c↓ 1.5 – 2 %)			
Improves glucose sensitivity, glucose tolerance, peripheral glucose uptake, while decreasesing hepatic gluconeogenesis, intestinal absorption of glucose.			
metformin	GLUCOPHAGE	500 mg QAM Titrate Weekly Max 1,000 BID **CrCl < 30 avoid**	GI: **Abdominal cramping**, flatulence, Nausea, Anorexia, **Black Box**: Lactic acidosis **Monitor**: BG, A1c, B12
Avoid: iodinated contrast media			
DPP4- inhibitors (Dipeptidyl Peptidase 4) (A1c↓ 0.5 – 0.8 %)			
The enzyme DPP4 degrades two incretins, GLP-1 and glucose dependent insulinotropic peptides (GIP) known for increasing insulin release, suppressing glucagon release, and delaying gastric emptying. Thus, DPP4-inhibitors allow GLP-1 and GIP to exist			
linagliptin	TRADJENTA	5 mg daily No renal adjustment	Nasopharyngitis, URTI, UTIs, Peripheral edema
sitagliptin	JANUVIA	100 mg daily **CrCl 30-50: 50 mg** **CrCl < 30: 25 mg**	GI upsets Acute pancreatitis Hypersensitivity reactions
GLP-1 AGONIST (A1c↓ 0.5 – 1.1%)			
An incretin-hormone secreted by **intestinal L** cells in response to a meal. Improves insulin secretion while inhibiting glucagon secretion, anorectic effect (weight loss)			
liraglutide	VICTOZA SAXENDA	0.6 mg/day x 1 week 1.2 mg/day x 1 week 1.8 mg/day thereafter	Increase satiety, metallic taste, Nausea, Diarrhea **Black Box**: thyroid carcinomas **Monitor**: BG, A1c,
INSULINS			
Activates enzymes, promotes transport of monosaccharide, facilitates the transformation of intracellular amino acids into proteins. All patient should be counseled on Sy/Sx and treatment of hypoglycemia.			
lispro	HUMALOG	Start 0.1-0.2 U/kg/day	**Hypoglycemia:** Sweating, Shaking, Dizziness, Jittery/Palpitation, Lightheadedness, Numbness, Nausea, Vomiting
aspart	NOVOLOG	Rapid Acting Bolus **(15 min before meal)**	
regular (human)	HUMULIN R	Start 0.1-0.2 U/Kg/day Short Acting Bolus **(30 min before meal)**	
detemir	LEVEMIR	50 % of Total Daily Dose	
glargine	LANTUS TOUGEO	Long Acting (Basal)	
Counseling on hypoglycemia: 15 g simple sugar 3-4 Glucose tablets, ½ cup (4 Oz) orange juice, full fat milk **Eat a snack** of slow-digesting carbs, whole grain crackers, bread, or cereal			

TABLE 2.2: ANTIDIABETICS

Medication Name		DOSING	ADVERSE REACTION
generic	**BRAND®**		
SGLT-2 Sodium-Glucose CO-Transporter 2 (A1c↓ 0.7 – 1 %)			
Inhibiting SGLT-2 in the proximal renal tubules, reduces reabsorption of filtered glucose from the tubular lumen into the blood circulations.			
canagliflozin	INVOKANA	100-300 mg/day before first meal, **CrCl 45-59: 100 mg** **CrCL < 45: avoid**	Infections (UTI, VVC) weight loss, urination, thirst **Monitor:** BG, A1c, BUN, Scr, Electrolytes, Fluid status **Boxed:** Increased amputations
SULFONYLUREA (A1c↓ 1 - 2%)			
Secretagogues block ATP-sensitive K⁺ channel, leads to depolarization and influx of Ca++ which results in insulin secretions from beta cells. Sometimes known as "oral insulins" for their "insulin like" side effects.			
glipizide	GLUCOTROL	2.5 – 20 mg daily, BID **for 10 Years** **No renal issue**	Hypoglycemia, **Weight gain** Nausea, Heartburn
glyburide	DIABETA MICRONASE GLUCOVANCE	1.25-20mg daily, BID **CrCl < 50: avoid**	Dizziness, B-cell burnout **Caution:** G6PD deficiency , **glimepiride** SJS, anaphylaxis **Monitor:** BG, A1c, Weight
glimepiride	AMARYL	1-8mg daily	
THIAZOLIDINEDIONES TZDs (A1c↓ 0.5 – 1.4 %)			
Sensitizer. Bind to nuclear transcription factors (PPARγ agonists) involved in insulin action. **Improves:** peripheral insulin sensitivity, insulin resistance, glucose uptake and utilization by peripheral tissues **decreases:** hepatic gluconeogenesis.			
pioglitazone	ACTOS	15-45 mg daily	Edema, Weight gain, Bladder Cancer, increased risk of limb fractures (myalgia) **CI:** CHF NYHA Class 3,4 **Monitor:** BG, A1c, LFTs
COMBINATIONS			
sitagliptin/ metformin	JANUMET (XR)	DPP4/ Biguanide	Constipation, Dry mouth, Stomach Pain Hypoglycemia, Weight gain, Lactic acidosis
****glipizide/ metformin**	METAGLIP	Sulfonyurea/ Biguanide	
****glyburide/ metformin**	GLUCOVANCE	Sulfonylurea/ Biguanide	

TABLE 2.3: CONTRACEPTIVES

Medication Name		DESCRIPTION	ADVERSE REACTION
generic	BRAND®		
Estrogens suppress Luteinizing hormone (LH), Follicle stimulation hormone (FSH), thickens cervical mucus, alters endometrium Progestin Only: **Progestins** suppresses ovulation, thickens cervical mucus, lower the midcycle of LH and FSH,			
norethindrone	ORTHO MICRONOR HEALTHER	Fixed dose of norethindrone (no placebo days)	Menstrual bleeding, Cramping (tender breasts) Leg Pain
desogestrel/ ethinyl estradiol (EE)	DESOGEN, ORTHO-CEPT, APRI	Active tables are taken **daily for 21 days**, followed by **inactive tablets for 7 days**. (21/7)	Abdominal pain cramping Chest pain or heaviness Headaches Eye or blurry vision Swelling or leg pain
drospirenone/ EE	YASMIN, OCELLA		
levonorgestrel/ EE	ALESSE, AVIANE, PORTIA, LEVO		
norgestimate/ EE	ORTHO-CYCLEN SPRINTEC		Serious: Cardiovascular Thrombosis (DVT/PE) Breakthrough bleeding
norethindrone/ EE/ FE	LOESTRIN FE, YAZ	24 active/ 4 inactive pill pack	
norgestimate/ EE (triphasic)	ORTHO TRI-CYCLEN TRISPRINTEC	Triphasic (7/7/7)	
norgestimate/ EE	OVRA, LO-OVRAL, OGESTREL	One tablet daily for 21 days only. No tablets for 7 days.	
medroxyprogester one	PROVERA	Inject every 3 months (150 mg IM or 104 mg SC)	Jaundice, cervical erosion/
	Black Box: All estrogen-containing products avoid use in women > 35 years old who smoke		
HORMONES			
Estradiol promotes growth of vagina, uterus, fallopian tubes, as well as stimulates RNA and protein synthesis to reduce hot flashes, vaginal dryness.			
estradiol patch	VIVELLE-DOT	0.025, 0.0375, 0.05, 0.075 or 1 mg per day patch	Edema, thrombosis
estrogens (conjugated)	PREMARIN tablet	0.3, 0.45, 0.625, 0.9, 1.25 mg	Bleeding, Jaundice
progesterone cap	PROMETRIUM	200 mg for 12 days sequentially per 28-day cycle at bedtime	Thromboembolic disorders, Blurry or loss of vision
estrogens (Conjugated) /medroxyprogeste rone	ACTIVELLA, FEMHRT, PREMPRO	Prempro 0.3 mg/1.5 mg, 0.625 mg/ 5 mg, etc.	Bleeding, Jaundice

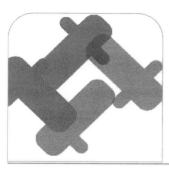

Table 3: Infectious Disease Medications

TABLE 3.1: ANTIBACTERIALS (See Dosing on Table 3.3-3.9)

Medication Name			
generic	**BRAND®**	**DRUG CLASS**	**ADVERSE REACTION**

CELL WALL SYNTHESIS INHIBITORS

Penicillins and Cephalosporins block the last step of bacterial cell wall synthesis called transpeptidation (cross linking) by binding to one or more penicillin-binding proteins (PBSs). **Time dependent, irreversible, bactericidal and beta-lactams.**

generic	BRAND®	DRUG CLASS	ADVERSE REACTION
cefdinir Tab,	OMNICEF	3rd gen Cephalosporin	GI upset, diarrhea, rash, cross sensitivity with PCN allergy, intestinal nephritis, myelosuppression, increase LFTs, seizures (conc. Based) **Monitor:** CBC, LFTs, Renal functions, anaphylaxis
cefprozil Tab,	CEFZIL	2nd Cephalosporin	
cefuroxime Tab,	CEFTIN	2nd gen Cephalosporin	
cephalexin Tab,	KEFLEX	1st gen cephalosporin	
amoxicillin Tab	AMOXIL, MOXATAG	Aminopenicillin	GI upset, diarrhea, rash, allergic reactions, seizures (conc. based)
amox-clav	AUGMENTIN		
penicilin VK Tablet, Susp	PEN-VEE K VEETIDS	Natural penicillin	**Monitor**: Bun/SCr, LFTs, CBC anaphylaxis

PROTEIN SYNTHESIS INHIBITORS

Tetracyclines binds to 30S and possibly 50s ribosomal subunits. They inhibit protein synthesis in a **bacteriostatic** fashion by blocking tRNA. Macrolides and Lincosamide binds to 50S subunit and indirectly block peptidyl transferase activity (A-P translocation and A-site binding). **bacteriostatic.**

generic	BRAND®	DRUG CLASS	ADVERSE REACTION
doxycycline tab, cap, susp, inj.	VIBRAMYCIN	Tetracycline	N/V/D rash, teeth discoloration, photosensitivity, skin reactions (SJS/TEN)
minocycline cap, tab, inj,	MINOCIN	Tetracycline	**Monitor:** LFTs, BUN/SCr, CBC
azithromycin tab, inj. susp. opth.	ZITHROMAX	Macrolide	Diarrhea, abd pain, cramping, severe skin reactions, QT prolongation,
clarithromycin tab, susp,	BIAXIN (XL)	Macrolide	**contraindication:** Hx of hepatic dysfunctions
clindamycin oral, Inj	CLEOCIN	Lincosamide	Severe diarrhea, urticaria, **Black Box:** colitis (C.*difficile*)
mupirocin topical, nasal	BACTROBAN		Burning, Local irritation, Rhinitis, Pharyngitis

Mupirocin inhibits bacterialisoleucyl transfer-RNA synthetase. A good mnemonic is "BUY AT $30, CCell $50" Aminoglycosides and Tetracyclines AT 30, Clindamycin, Erythromycin (Macrolides), Lincomycin, Linezolid AT 50.

TABLE 3.2: ANTIBACTERIALS (CONT.)

Medication Name		DRUG CLASS	ADVERSE REACTION
generic	BRAND®		
DNA/ RNA INHIBITORS			
Quinolones inhibit DNA gyrase, the enzyme that regulates supercoiling of DNA. Also, inhabit topoisomerase IV, the enzyme that separates interlinked DNA after replication. They are bactericidal			
ciprofloxacin tab, susp, Inj, oint, otic	CIPRO	Quinolones	Nausea, Diarrhea, Headache, Insomnia, AKI, QT prolongation, Photosensitivity, avoid chelators **Boxed: Tendon rupture** **Monitor:** CBC, Renal and Liver function
levofloxacin tab, susp, Inj, ophthalmic	LEVAQUIN	Quinolones	
ofloxacin	OCUFLOX	Quinolones	
NITROFURANS			
Inhibits bacterial enzymes, acetyl Co-A and damages their DNA. They are bactericidal at high conc.			
nitrofurantoin cap, susp	MACROBID MACRODANTIN	Nitrofuran **CrCl < 60 avoid**	GI upset, fever, chill, brown urine **take with food, G6PD issues**
metronidazole tab, cap, inj	FLAGYL	Nitroimidazole	Seizures, nausea, metallic test, darkened urine, SJS, seizures, neuropathies.
ANTI-METABOLITES			
Decreases bacterial folic acid synthesis by competitively inhibiting dihydropteroate synthase. Sulfonamides are **bactericidal**			
sulfamethoxazole trimethoprim	BACTRIM SEPTRA	Anti-metabolites	Diarrhea, Rash, skin reaction, anorexia, crystalluria, hypoglycemia, myelosuppression, photosensitivity, SJS/ TEN
		Monitoring: CBC, Renal, LFTs, Folate **Contraindications:** Sulfa allergy	
OTHER AGENTS			
chlorhexidine	PERIDEX	Antiplaque	Alteration of taste, mouth irritation
bacitracin/neomycin/polymyxin B topical, ophthalmic	NEO-POLYCIN NEOSPORIN	Aminoglycosides (neomycin) in combination	Pruritus, erythema, anaphylactoid reaction
Chlorhexidine disruption of plasma membrane of bacterial cell, Bacitracin is a bacteriostatic, cell wall inhibitor; Neomycin is an aminoglycoside, and Polymxin B is a cell membrane inhibitor			

TABLE 3.3: ANTIFUNGALS, ANTIVIRALS, ANTIPARASITIC

Medication Name		DRUG CLASS	ADVERSE REACTION
generic	BRAND®		
ANTIFUNGALS			
Decrease ergosterol synthesis and inhibit cell membrane formation.			
fluconazole tab, susp, inj	DIFLUCAN	Azoles	Abdominal Pain, Diarrhea Rash, QT prolongation, hypertension, edema, hair loss or gain. **Boxed:** ketoconazole hepatotoxicity
ketoconazole tab, cream, foam, gel, shampoo	NIZORAL	Azoles	
terbinafine tab, granule, topical	LAMISIL	Other antifungal agents	Headache, Diarrhea, abdominal pain, dyspepsia, nystatin: (Burning, itching, rash)
nystatin topical	NYSTOP		
		Contraindications: liver disease: **Monitor:** LFTs, Lipids, EKG, CBC	
acyclovir cap, tab, buccal, susp, inj, topical	ZOVIRAX	DNA polymerase inhibitor	Malaise, Headache, N/V/D rash, pruritus, seizures, burning
valacyclovir tab, susp,	VALTREX		Fever, N/V/D, anorexia, thrombocytopenia, neutropenia, anemia, seizures, retinal detachment
		Black: Myelosupression **Monitoring:** CBC with differential, PL SCr, Retinal exam, Renal function, LFTs, CBC, SCr/BUN	
emtricitabine tenofovir disoproxil elvitegravir, cobicistat	STRIBILD	2 NRTIs+INSTIs **CrCL < 70: avoid**	Insomnia, diarrhea, rash, dreams **Black box:** Lactic acidosis **Monitoring:** CPK, LFTs, Renal **take with food, avoid chelators**
oseltamivir	TAMIFLU	Neuraminidase inhibitors **CrCL ≤ 60: adjust**	Headache, N/V/D, abdominal pain, hallucination, delirium, SJS
		Reduce the amount of virus in the body by inhibiting the release of new viral particles	
ANTIPARASITIC			
Increase membrane permeability (permeating the chitin of the fungal cell wall)			
**permethrin	ELIMITE		Stinging, Erythema, Irritation of the skin

TABLE 3.4: DOSAGE RECOMMENDATIONS TO ANTIMICROBIALS

NOTE: Dosing recommendations vary depending on indication. Refer to package insert for full information.

ANTIBIOTIC	USUAL DOSE	RENAL DOSE	HEMODIALYSIS
acyclovir	IV: 5-20 mg/kg q8h PO:200-800mg q6-8h	25-100: dose q12h 10-25: dose q24h <10: 50% of dose q24h	2.5-5 mg/kg/24hr (40-50% dialyzable)
amikacin	IV/IM: 5-7.5 mg/kg q8h OR 15-20 mg/kg/day	40-60: q12h 20-40: q12h	5-7.5 mg/kg q48-72h individualized (20% dialyzable)
amoxicillin	PO: 250-500 mg q8h 500-875 mg BID	10-30: 250-500 mg q12h <10: 250-500 q24h	250-500 daily (avoid ER tabs) 875 mg IR
amox/clav	PO: 250-500 mg q8h 875 mg q12h	<30: avoid 875 mg or ER tab 10-30: 250-500 mg q12h <10: 250-500 mg q24h	250-500 mg q24h after dialysis 875 mg IR (avoid ER tabs)
amphotericin	IV: 0.5-1 mg/kg/day	50% of dose on alternate dates	Poorly dialyzed
amphotericin lipid	IV:3-6 mg/kg/day	No renal adjustment needed	No evidence
ampicillin	IV:1-2 g q4-6h PO: 250-500 mg q6h	>50: q4-6h 10-50: q6-12h <10: q12-24h	No evidence
ampicillin	IV: 1-2 g q4-6h PO: 250-500 mg q6h	>50: q4-6h 10-50: q6-12h <10: q12-24h	1-2 g q12-24h after dialysis (20-50% dialyzable)
ampicillin/sulbactam	IV: 1.5-3 g q6h	15-30: 1.5-3 g q12h 5-14: 1.5-3 g q24h	1.5-3g q12-24 after dialysis
azithromycin	250-500 mg q24h	CrCl <10 avoid	No evidence

TABLE 3.5: DOSAGE RECOMMENDATIONS TO ANTIMICROBIALS

ANTIBIOTIC	USUAL DOSE	RENAL DOSE	HEMODIALYSIS
aztreonam	IV: 1-2 g q6-8h	10-30: 50 % of usual dose	**Loading Dose**: 500 mg 2 g, then 25 % of initial dose at usual interval (20-50 % dialyzable)
cefazolin	IV: 1-2 g q6-8h	25-60: Full dose in intervals > 8 h 11-34: 50% of usual dose q 12 h	500 mg 1 g q24h or 1-2g q48-72h (20-50% dialyzable)
cefidinir	PO: 300 mg BID 600 mg q24h	<30: 300 mg q24h	HD: 300 mg q48h with 300 mg post-HD PD: same dose for CrCl <10
cefepime	IV: 1-2 g q8-12h	30-60: 0.5-2 g q12-24h 11-29: 0.5-2 g q24h <11: 0.25-1 g q24h	1 g on day 1; then 0.5-1 g q24h 1-2g q48-72h 2g 3 times weekly after dialysis
cefepime PK dosing	IV: 1 g q6h	30-50: 1g q8h 15-29: 1 g q12h <15: 1 g24h	
cefotaxime	IV: 1-2 g q 4-12h	10-50: q6-12h <10: q48h	Administer 1-2 g q24h
cefotetan	IV: 0.5-3 g q12h	10-30: q24h <10: q48h	25% of dose q24h on non-dialysis days 50% dose on dialysis day (5-20% dialyzable)
cefoxitin	IV: 1-2 g q6-8h	30-50: 1-2 g q8-12h 10-29: 1-2 g q12-24h 5-9: 0.5 1 g q12-24h <5: 0.5-1 g q24-48h	LD: 1-2 g after each HD sessions

TABLE 3.6: DOSAGE RECOMMENDATIONS TO ANTIMICROBIALS

ANTIBIOTIC	USUAL DOSE	RENAL DOSE	HEMODIALYSIS
ciprofloxacin	IV: 400 mg q8-12h PO: 250-500 mg BID	IV: 5-29: 200-400 mg q18-24h PO:30-50: 250-500 mg q12h 5-29: 250-500 mg q12h	200-400 mg q24h (dialyzable < 10%)
clarithromycin	PO: 250-500 mg q12h	<30: decrease dose by 50%	Give after HD
clindamycin	PO: 150-450 mg q6h PO: Max: 1.8 g daily IV: 600-1200 mg daily in 2-4 divided doses IV Max: 4.8 g daily	No dose adjustment needed	No dose adjustment needed
colistin	IV: 2.5-5 mg/kg/day 2-4 doses	50-79: 2.5-3.8 mg/kg/day BID 30-49: 2.5 mg/kg/day daily or BID 10-29: 1.5 mg/kg q36h	1.5 mg/kg q24-48h after dialysis
dalbavancin	IV:1000mg on day 1, then 500 mg on day 8 OR 1500 mg single dose	<30: 750 mg on day 1, then 375 mg on day 8 OR 1125 mg as a single dose	No dose adjustment needed
daptomycin	IV: 4-8 mg/kg q24h	<30: extend interval to q48h	Administer 3 times weekly (50% dialyzable)
doxycycline	IV/PO: 100-200 mg/day in 1-2 divided doses	No adjustment needed	No adjustment needed
ertapenem	IV/IM: 1 g daily	<30: 500mg daily	If given > 6 h prior no adjustment needed; if within 6 hours give 150 mg
erythromycin	IV: 3mg/kg over 45 min q8h PO: 250-500 mg q6-12h	No evidence	5-20% dialyzable

TABLE 3.7: DOSAGE RECOMMENDATION TO ANTIMICROBIALS

ANTIBIOTIC	USUAL DOSE	RENAL DOSE	HEMODIALYSIS
famciclovir	PO: 250-500 mg q8-12h	40-59: 500 mg q12h 20-39: 500 mg q24h <20: 250 mg q24h	125-250 mg after dialysis
fluconazole	IV/PO: 150 mg once or LD: 200-800 mg Maintenance: 200-800 mg daily	≤50: Decrease dose by 50%	No dose adjustment needed
fosfomycin	PO: 3 g	No evidence	No evidence
ganciclovir	iv: 5 mg/kg q12-24h (maintenance)	50-69 2.5 mg/kg/dose q24h 25-49: 1.25mg/kg/dose q24h 10-24: 0.625 mg/kg/dose q24h	0.625 mg/kg q48-72h (50% dialyzable)
gemifloxacin	PO: 320 mg daily	<40: 160 mg daily	160 mg daily after HD
gentamicin	IV/IM 1-2.5 mg/kg q8-12h **OR** 4-7 mg/kg/dose/day	40-60: q12h 20-40: q24h	LD: 2-3mg/kg → 1-2 mg/kg q48-72h) (50% dialyzable)
imipenem	IV:250-1000 mg q6-8h	<70 adjust dose	after HD and q12h after
isavuconazole	IV/PO: LD 200 mg q8h for 48h Maintenance: 200 mg q24h	No evidence	No evidence
itraconazole	PO: 200-400 mg daily	No evidence	No evidence
levofloxacin	IV/PO: 500 -750 mg q24h	LD + 250 – 500 q48h	LD+ 250 – 500 mg q48h
linezolid	IV/PO: 600mg BID	No dose adjustment needed	after dialysis

TABLE 3.8: DOSAGE RECOMMENDATIONS TO ANTIMICROBIALS

ANTIBIOTIC	USUAL DOSE	RENAL DOSE	HEMODIALYSIS
meropenem	IV: 1.5-6g daily divided q6-8h	26-50: q12h 10-25: 50% of dose q12h <10: 50% of dose q24h	500 mg q 24h (dialyzable)
meropenem PK dosing	IV: 500 mg q6h	26-50: 500 mg q8h 10-25: 500 mg q12h <10: 500 mg q24h	No evidence
metronidazole	IV/PO: 250-750 mg q6-8h	No dose adjustment needed	500 mg q8-12h (50-100% dialyzable)
minocycline	IV/PO: 200 mg → 100 mg q12h	No dose adjustment needed	<80: max 200 mg
moxifloxacin	IV/PO: 50-100 mg q6-12h	<40 mg/min: avoid	<40mg/min avoid
nitrofurantoin	PO: 50-100 mg q6-12h	<40: avoid	<40 avoid
oritavancin	IV: 1200 mg	No evidence	No evidence
oseltamivir	PO: 75-100 mg BID	30-60: 30 mg BID 10-30: 30 mg once daily	30 mg post dialysis
Pipercillin/ Tazobactam	IV: 3.375-4.5 g q6-8h	20-40: 3.375 g q8h <20: 3.375 g q12h	2.25g q12h
Pipercillin/tazo PK dosing	IV: 3.375 g q8h → 4hrs	<20: 3.375 g q12h → 4h	No evidence
posaconazole	IV: 300 mg q12h day 1 → 300 mg daily PO: 200 mg q8h with food	IV: <50 avoid IV: <20 no evidence	No evidence

TABLE 3.9: DOSAGE RECOMMENDATIONS TO ANTIMICROBIALS

ANTIBIOTIC	USUAL DOSE	RENAL DOSE	HEMODIALYSIS
rifampin	TB: IV/PO: 10 mg /kg q24h Meningitis: 600 mg q24h	No dose adjustment necessary	No dose adjustment necessary
Sulfamethoxazole/ trimethoprim	IV: 8-20 mg TMP/kg/day q6-12h PO: 1-2 800/160mg q12-24h	15-30: 50% of dose	2.5-10 mg/kg TMP q24h or 20mg/kg TMP 3x/week after HD
Tedizolid	IV/PO: 200 mg once daily	No dose adjustment necessary	No dose adjustment needed
Televancin	IV: 10 mg/kg/day	31-50: 7.5mg kg q24h 10-30: 10 mg/kg q48h	No evidence
Tetracycline	PO: 250-500 mg q6h	50-80: q8-12h 10-50: q12-24h, <10: q24h	q24h (5-20% dialyzable)
tigecycline	IV: LD 100 mg Maintenance: 50 mg q12h	No dose adjustment needed	No dose adjustment needed
tobramycin	IV/IM: 1-2.5 mg/kg q8-12h **Or** 4-7 mg/kg/dose daily	40-60: q12h 20-40: q24h, <20: LD then monitor	LD: 2-3 mg/kg → 1-2 mg/kg 48-72h (50% dialyazable)
valacyclovir	PO: 0.5-2 g q6-24h	30-49: 1 g q12h 10-29: 1 g24h<10: 500 mg q24h	After hemodialysis (30% dialyzable)
valganciclovir	PO: 900 mg BID	40-59: 450 mg BID 25-39: 450 mg daily 10-24: 450 mg q48h	avoid: 100-200 mg 3x post HD
vancomycin	IV: 15-20 mg /kg/dose q8-12h PO: 125-500 q6h	IV: 20-49: 750-1500 mg q24h <20 refer to trough	LD: 15-25 mg/kg → 0.5-1 g or 5-10 mg/kg post HD sessions (30-50% dialyzable)
voriconazole	IV: 6mg/kg BID 2 doses maintenance: 4 mg/k	no evidence	no evidence

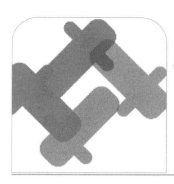

Table 4: GI and Dietary Disorders

TABLE 4.1: ANTIHYPERLIPIDEMIC

Medication Name		DOSING	DRUG INTERACTIONS
GENERIC	BRAND		
atorvastatin	LIPITOR	40-80 mg Daily High 10-20 mg daily moderate	avoid cyclosporine, gemfibrozil max 40mg: ritonavir+saquinavir
rosuvastatin	CRESTOR	20-40 mg High 5-10 mg daily moderate **CrCL < 30 avoid**	max 5 mg: cyclosporin, warfarin (levels) max 10 mg: gemfibrozil, protease inhibitor.
lovastatin	MEVACOR	20-40 mg daily Moderate 20 mg daily low **CrCL < 30 avoid**	avoid strong 3A4s plus tacrolimus max 20mg: danazol, diltiazem, verapamil, amlodipine max 40 mg: amiodarone, ticagrelor
pravastatin	PRAVACHOL	40-80 mg daily Moderate 10-20 mg daily low **CrCL < 60 avoid**	max 20 mg: cyclosporine max 40 mg: clarithromycin
simvastatin	ZOCOR	20-40 mg daily Moderate 10 mg daily low **CrCL < 30 avoid**	avoid strong 3A4s plus conivaptan, tacrolimus max 10 mg: verapamil, diltiazem max 20 mg: amiodarone, amlodipine,
Side Effects include: Myalgia, Arthralgias, Myopathy, Diarrhea, Cognitive impairment **CI:** liver disease, pregnancy, breastfeeding **Monitoring: LFT (Liver Panel)**			
OTHER AGENTS			
fenofibrate	TRICOR	48-145 mg daily **CrCL 30-80 low dose**	
gemfibrozil	LOPID	600 mg BID **CrCL < 30 avoid**	Avoid ezetimibe or statins
Dyspepsia, Abdominal Pain, Rash, Muscle Pain, Tenderness, Weakness **CONTRAINDICATIONS:** biliary cirrhosis **Monitor:** LFTs, CPK, CrCL			
omega-3-acid	LOVAZA	Refer to labeling	Belching, Taste disturbance, Infection symptoms
niacin	NIASPAN	500 mg HS increase wkly (IR vs ER)	Take niacin 4-6 hours after bile acid sequestrants
ezetimibe	ZETIA	10 mg daily	Monitor levels of cyclosporine
**ezetimibe/ simvastatin	VYTORIN	**CrCL < 60 low dose**	Monitor levels of cyclosporine
MOA: Inhibition of cholesterol absorption **AE:** Diarrhea, URTIs, arthralgias, myalgias			

TABLE 4.2: LAXATIVES, and ANTIDIARRHEA

Medication Name		DOSING	ADVERSE REACTION
GENERIC	**BRAND**		
**linaclotide cap	LINZESS	PO: 145 mcg daily IBS dosing 290 mcg	Diarrhea, flatulence, headache **Contraindication:** Age < 6; GI obstruction
MOA: An agonist of guanylate cyclase C, help reduce GI transit time by increasing chloride and bicarbonate secretion. **Boxed:** Dehydration, avoid in pediatrics			
docusate sodium cap, enema, syrup	COLASE	PO: 50 – 360 daily Enema: 283 g/5 mL	Abdominal cramping **Contraindication:** Abdominal pain
MOA: Emollient, help soften the surface tension of the oil/water composition of stool **Onset:** 12 to 72 hours, preferred in postpartum, MI, anal fissures, hemorrhoids			
PEG 3350	MIRALAX GLYCOLAX GOLYTELY	17 g in 4-8 oz of beverage. Max 100 grams/day.	Electrolyte imbalance, gas, dehydration, **Contraindication:** GI obstruction
MOA: Osmotic laxative, help retain fluid in the bowel lumen increasing peristalsis. Golytely is used for Bowel Prep. Take with water			
diphenoxylate/ atropine sulfate C-V	LOMOTIL	5 – 20 mg daily	Constipation, Dry mouth, Stomach pain
MOA: Diphenoxylate binds to intestinal opiate receptors decreasing peristalsis and affecting water/electrolyte movement. Atropine discourage abuse/overdose			
mesalamine (5-ASA) tab, cap, supp	LIALDA PENTASA CANASA	refer to literature for dosing	Abdominal pain, Nausea, Headache, Flatulence, Belching (eructation) pharyngitis
MOA: Aminosalicylate an anti-inflammatory **Contraindication:** Hypersensitivity **Monitor:** Bun/SrCr, CBC			
dicyclomine	BENTYL	10 mg daily	Stomach pain, Heartburn, Reflux, anticholinergic effects
MOA: Blocks the action of acetylcholine at parasympathetic sites in smooth muscles. **Monitor:** Urinary output			

TABLE 4.3: ELECTROLYTES, and SUPPLEMENTS

Medication Name		DOSING	ADVERSE REACTION
GENERIC	**BRAND**		
magnesium chloride tab	MgCL	Male: 400-420 mg daily Female: 310 mg daily	Respiratory depression, Flushing, Hypotension, Sweating
	Drug Interactions: doxycycline, minocycline tetracycline **Monitor**: CBC (Glucose, K+), EKG		
potassium chloride IV, tap, cap, bulk	KLOR-CON, K-DUR	10-100 mEq daily	Abdominal discomfort, N/V, Flatulence
	Contraindication: Hyperkalemia, Pregnancy C **Monitor**: CBC (Glucose, K+), EKG		
VITAMINS AND SUPPLEMENTS			
folic acid IV, tab	FOLIC ACID	1 mg daily	Hypersensitivity reaction
	Drug Interactions: fosphenytoin, methotrexate, phenobarbital, phenytoin		
calcitriol oral, cap	ROCALTROL	0.25 mcg Dialysis: 0.25 mcg daily	Weakness, headache, somnolence, N/V dry mouth muscle pain, metallic taste
	MOA: Synthetic vitamin D analog (1α,25-dihydroxy-cholecalcifero) active in the absorption of Ca+ from the GI tract. **Warnings**: Hypercalcemia, Ca+ intoxication **Monitor**: Ca+ levels, Phosphate,/ PTH levels		
cyanocobalamin (B-12) inj, sublingual	B-12 INJECTION NASCOBAL	IM: 1,000 mcg daily → 7 days, weekly → 1 month → monthly 6 months	Skin rash, Diarrhea, Hypokalemia, thrombosis, hypersensitivity, edema
	MOA: Coenzyme for various metabolic activities.		
ergocalciferol (D3) oral, tab	DRISDOL	see literature for dosing	Constipation, Bone demineralization, Weight loss
	MOA: Vitamin D_2 is a provitamin, the active metabolite (calcitriol) stimulates calcium and phosphate absorption.		
ferrous sulfate oral, syrup, tab	FER-IN-SOL FEROSUL	see literature for dosing	Darkening of stool, Abdominal pain, Heartburn, Flatulence
	MOA: Replace iron found in hemoglobin **Monitor**: RBC, Hemoglobin, Hematocrit		

TABLE 4.4: ANTIEMETICS, ANTISECRETORY AND WEIGHT LOSS

Medication Name			
generic	**BRAND®**	**DOSING**	
5-HT3 RECEPTOR ANTAGONIST			
ondansetron HCL IV, oral	ZOFRAN	refer to literature	Fatigue, Constipation, Headache
metoclopramide IV, oral	REGLAN	10-15mg daily	Restlessness, Tardive Dyskinesia, Drowsiness, Restlessness, Fatigue, Diarrhea
promethazine IV, oral, rectal	PHENERGAN	refer to literature	Blurry vision, Dry mouth, Rash
famotidine Tab, Chew, Susp, Inj	PEPCID	10-20 MG BID PRN **CrCL< 50: 5 mg**	Dizziness, Headache, Stomach problems, QT prolongation (famotidine)
ranitidine Tab, Chew, Susp, Inj, Syrup	ZANTAC	75-150 mg BID PRN	
	Onset: within 60 minutes so take 30-60 minutes before food that cause heart burn **Duration**: 4-10 hours **Monitor:** ECG changes, ALT		
dexlansoprazole Cap, ODT	DEXILANT	30-60 mg daily	
lansoprazole Cap, ODT, SUSP	PREVACID	15-30 mg daily	Abdominal Pain Flatulence
esomeprazole Cap, Inj, Packet	NEXIUM	20-40 mg daily **No renal adjustment**	Headache Nausea Diarrhea (mild)
omeprazole Tab, Cap, Packet	Prilosec	20 mg daily	Skin reaction with IV PROTONIX
pantoprazole Tab, Inj, Packet	PROTONIX	40 mg daily	
	MOA: Suppress H/K ATPase **Onset:** 1-3 hours with **duration** > 24 hours May be used in pregnancy. Mix but not crush capsules		
phentermine Cap, tab	ADIPEX-P LONAMIN	37.6 mg daily CrCl 15-30: 15 mg daily Take prior to breakfast	Constipation, diarrhea, restlessness, taste disturbances
	MOA: Sympathomimetic amine (CNS stimulation/ elevation of BP) **Contraindication:** age <16, long term use		

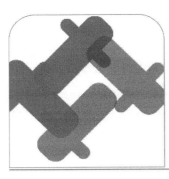

Table 5: Musculoskeletal Seizure and Pain Disorders

TABLE 5.1: ANALGESICS and OPIOIDS

Medication Name		DOSING	ADVERSE REACTION
generic	BRAND®	DOSING	ADVERSE REACTION
lidocaine topical	LIDODERM	apply thin film	Localized burning, Dermatitis
	MOA: Stabilizes neuronal membrane by inhibiting Na channel repolarization		
betamethasone/ clotrimazole topical	LOTRISONE	apply thin film	Localized burning
	MOA: Betamethasone is a corticosteroid, clotrimazole is an antifungal.		
tramadol	Ultram Ultracet	IR: 50-100 mg q4-6h ER: 100 mg daily CrCL <30: max 200mg	Constipation, Dizziness, Nausea, Somnolence (Drowsiness)
	MOA: Binds to μ-opioid receptor, inhibits reuptake of NE and serotonin reuptake. **Contraindication:** use in children <12 years		
butalbital/APAP/ caffeine	FIORICET	fixed dose	Dizziness, Somnolence
	Acetaminophen inhibits prostaglandin synthesis		

OPIOIDS

MOA: Opioid Analgesic, interact with central opioid receptors.

generic	BRAND®	DOSING	ADVERSE REACTION
hydrocodone bitartrate /acetaminophen	LORTAB VICODIN	5-10 mg/ 325 mg, q6h	Constipation, Drowsiness, Sweating, Dizziness, lightheadedness, side effects related to acetaminophen
oxycodone/ acetaminophen	ENDOCET PERCOCET	IR: 5-20 mg q4-6h CR: 10-80 mg	
**codeine/ acetaminophen	TYLENOL (#2, 3, 4)	200-400 mg q4-6h, PRN	**Boxed:** Respiratory depression, Ultra-rapid metabolizers of codeine (2D6 polymorphism) in codeine and CYP3A4 inhibitors in fentanyl and oxycodone.
morphine sulfate ER tab, cap, inj, supp, soln	MS CONTIN	IR: 10-30 mg q4h, prn ER: 15-200 q6-12h	
hydromorphone tab, inj, soln	DILAUDID DILAUDID HP	PO: 2-4 mg q4-6h, PRN IV: 0.2-1 mg, q2-3h	
**oxymorphone	OPANA	IR: 5-10mg q4-6h PRN	**Monitoring:** BP, Pain Scale
oxycodone	OXYCONTIN ROXYBOND	IR: 5-20 mg q4-6h CR: 10-80 q12h	**Counseling:** Habit forming, do not crush CR, avoid alcohol, take with full glass of water
**methadone	METHADONE	2.5-10 mg q6-12h	
fentanyl (transdermal)	DURAGESIC	1 patch q48-72h	

TABLE 5.1: NON-OPIOID AND ANTIANXIETY

Medication Name		DOSING	ADVERSE REACTION
generic	BRAND®		
buprenorphine/ naloxone buccal film, patch, tab, sublingual	SUBOXONE ZUBSOLV	refer to literature	Sedation, Dizziness, Headache, Confusion, QT Prolongation
	MOA: buprenorphine is a partial mu-opioid agonist, naloxone is an opioid antagonist. **Boxed:** Risk of addiction abuse, and misuse.		
epinephrine auto-injector	EpiPen	refer to literature	Sweating, Respiratory problems, Anxiety Weakness, Palpitation
	MOA: Acts on alpha and beta receptors leading to loss of intravascular volume, muscle relaxation		
acetaminophen tab, cap, chew, ODT, susp, supp, inj	TYLENOL OFIRMEV	refer to literature max < 4,000 mg/days	Skin rash **Boxed:** Severe hepatotoxicity
	MOA: non-opioid, non-anti-inflammatory analgesics. Works through inhibition of prostaglandin synthesis in the CNS, inhibition of N-methyl D-aspartate (NMDA)		
alprazolam tab, ODT, oral, soln	XANAX XANAX XR	0.25-0.5 TID	Somnolence (Drowsiness)
clonazepam tab, ODT	KLONOPIN	0.25-0.5 mg BID	Dizziness Weakness
diazepam	VALIUM	2-10 mg BID-QID	Ataxia (Impaired balance)
lorazepam tab, inj, oral, sol	ATIVAN LORAZEPAM	2-3 mg PO daily	Lightheadedness
temazepam	RESTORIL	15 to 30 mg at qHS	Drowsiness, lethargy, confusion
	MOA: interacts with GABA receptors. **Boxed:** Use with opioids increases sedation, respiratory depression **Contraindication:** sleep apnea, cirrhosis. Alprazolam with 3A4 inhibitors (azoles) **Counseling:** Avoid abrupt discontinuation if used for more than 10 days; habit forming.		
topiramate cap, tab	TOPAMAX TOPIRAGEN TROKENDI XR	refer to literature max 400 mg/day CrCl <70: 50% decrease	Somnolence, Dizziness Short term memory issue Weight loss **Contraindications:** alcohol use within 6h
	MOA: Blocks voltage-dependent Na+ channels, enhances GABAa activity, **Monitoring:** suicidal thoughts, intraocular pressure, serum, bicarbonate, renal functions **Counseling:** Drink plenty of fluid, can cause eye problems, blood acidity, decrease sweating,		
buspirone	BUSPAR	10-15 mg BID-TID **No renal adjustment**	Nausea, headache, Somnolence
	MOA: Acts on serotonin (5-HT1A and 5-HT2) receptors; moderate affinity for dopamine (D2)		

TABLE 5.2: ANTISEIZURE AGENTS

Medication Name			
generic	BRAND®	DOSING	ADVERSE REACTION
			ANTICONVULSANT
carbamazepine cap, tab, chew, ing, susp	TEGRETOL TEGRETOL XR	200 mg BID-QID max 1,600 mg QD **CrCl <60: avoid use**	Dizziness, Unsteadiness, N/V, Dry mouth, Pruritus, Alopecia, Decrease in bone density
	MOA: Na+ channel blocker **INDICATION:** Bipolar **Off-Label:** Neuralgia, pain **Monitoring/Level:** 4-12 mg/mL within 3-5days, CBC with differential/ platelets/ LFTs, D/C < 2,500 WBC< ANC < 1,000 **Counseling:** take with food		
divalproex	DEPAKOTE DEPAKOTE ER	10-15 mg/kg/day max: 60 mg/kg/qd **no renal adjustment**	Asthenia, Somnolence, Dyspepsia, Dose related thrombocytopenia
	MOA: increases GABA **Boxed:** Hepatic failure, fetal harm **Monitoring/Level:** LFTs, CBC w/diff, platelets **Counseling:** CBC w/platelets, PT/PTT,		
gabapentin	NEURONTIN	Initial dose of 300 mg daily-BID to dose of 600 mg TID, CrCl <60: 200-700 BID, CrCl<30 daily	Seizure, Mood, Brain, Possible abrupt cessation withdrawal
	MOA: Ca+ channel blocker, no GABA activity **INDICATION:** Neuropathic pain **Monitoring/Level:** suicidality		
lamotrigine	LAMICTAL LAMICTAL XR	refer to literature	Rash, Dizziness, Somnolence Drug interaction with valproic acid.
	MOA: Ca+ channel blocker, binds to GABA **Boxed: SJS/TEN**		
levetiracetam tab, soln, inj	KEPPRA KEPPRA XR	500 mg BID or XR: 1000 mg daily Max: 3,000 daily **CrCL≤80: low dose**	Somnolence, Asthenia, Dizziness, Mental issues with long term use,
	MOA: Na+ channel blocker, inhibits burst firing **Monitoring/Level:** **Counseling:** Do not chew break tablet		
oxcarbazepine	TRILEPTAL, OXTELLAR XR	300 mg BID XR 600 mg daily	Dizziness, Fatigue, SJS/TEN (HLAB*1502)
	MOA: Block Na channels **Monitoring/Level:** CBC, serum Na+		
pregabalin	LYRICA	seizures: 150 mg daily BID, TID –600 mg daily T2DM Neuropathy: 25 to 75 mg daily BID **CrCl <60:50% of usual**	Dizziness, Somnolence, Dry Mouth; Possible abrupt cessation withdrawal
	MOA: Ca+ Channel blocker, no GABA activity **INDICATION:** Neuropathic pain **Off-Label:** DM **Monitoring/Level:** **Counseling** Unknown (related to high binding affinity to alpha-2 delta site in CNS tissue		

TABLE 5.3: ANTISEIZURE AGENTS (CONT..)

Medication Name			
generic	BRAND®	DOSING	ADVERSE REACTION
		ANTICONVULSANT	
**phenobarbital	PHENOBARBITAL	50 – 100 mg BID	Somnolence, Cognitive impairment, Dizziness, Depression
MOA: Na+ channel blocker **Monitoring/Level:** 20-40 mcg/mL, LFTs, CBC with differential **Counseling**			
phenytoin cap, chew, susp, inj	DILANTIN	LD: 15—20 mg/Kg MD: 300-600 mg/day	Ataxia, Slurred speech, Mental issue, gingival hyperplasia, hair growth, hepatotoxicity
MOA: Na channel blocker **Boxed:** IV:50 mg/min **Monitoring/Level:** 10=20 mcg/mL			
primidone	MYSOLINE	refer to literature dose titration required. **CrCl 10-50: q12h**	Ataxia, Dizziness, Impotence, Rash, Nystagmus
MOA: decreases neuron excitability, raises seizure threshold, similar to phenobarbital. **Monitoring/Level:** serum primidone/ phenobarbital			
**zonisamide cap	ZONEGRAN	200 mg daily increase dose after 2 weeks **CrCl < 40 avoid**	Anorexia, Dizziness, dizziness, Irritability
MOA: inhibits Na+ and Ca+ channel, no GABA activity **Monitoring/Level:** BUN/SrCr, serum bicarbonate, suicidal thoughts			

TABLE 5.4: OSTEOPOROSIS AGENTS

Medication Name			
generic	BRAND®	DOSING	ADVERSE REACTION
alendronate tab, soln	FOSAMAX	10 mg daily, 70 mg wkly prevention 50% of usual **CrCl <35: avoid**	Abdominal pain, Hypocalcemia, hypophosphatemia, heartburn
MOA: inhibiting osteoclast activity. **Contraindication:** inability to sit-up for 30 min, osteonecrosis of the jaw			
raloxifene	EVISTA	60 mg daily	Hot flashes, Leg cramps, Peripheral edema, N/D
MOA: selective estrogen receptor modulator (SERM) **Boxed:** Endometrial cancer; VTE/Stroke			

TABLE 5.5: PAIN AGENTS

Medication Name			
generic	BRAND®	DOSING	ADVERSE REACTION
ANTISPASMODICS (MUSCLE RELAXANTS)			
baclofen tab, inj	LIORESAL	5-20 mg TID,QID,PRN	Drowsiness, Dizziness Weakness, Confusion
MOA: Produce smooth muscle relaxation **Boxed:** abrupt withdrawal of intrathecal			
carisoprodol CIV	SOMA	250-350 mg QID, PRN Low dose poor 2C19	Drowsiness, Dizziness
MOA: Unknown may produce smooth muscle relaxation by sedation.			
cyclobenzaprine tab, cap	FLEXERIL, AMRIX,	IR: 5-10 mg TID, PRN ER: 15-30 mg daily	Dry mouth, caution in elderly
MOA: Reduces tonic somatic motor activity			
methocarbamol tab, IV	ROBAXIN	500–2,000 mg daily	Pruritus, Rash, Hypotension, Drowsiness
MOA: Inhibiting flexor and crossed extensor reflexes			
**orphenadrine citrate	NORFLEX	Oral: 100 mg BID IM, IV: 60 mg q12h	Drowsiness, Dry mouth, Agitation, Pruritus, tachycardia
MOA: muscle relaxant by central atropine-like effect;			
tizanidine tab, cap	ZANAFLEX	2-4 mg q6-8h PRN	Drowsiness, Weakness, Abnormal LFT, Blurry vision
MOA: Alpha-2 adrenergic agonist, reduces spasticity inhibition of motor neurons			
COX-1 and COX-2 Non-Selective			
MOA: Inhibition of cyclooxygenase resulting in decreased prostaglandins (PG)			
ibuprofen tab, cap, chew, susp, inj	ADVIL MOTRIN	200 – 800 MG q6-8h ≤ 10days	Rash, Abdominal cramps
**indomethacin oral, cap, susp, inj	INDOCIN, TIVORBEX	IR 25-50 mg BID CR: 75 mg daily-BID	GI cramping, abdominal pain
naproxen	NAPROSYN	200-550 mg q8-12h	Shortness of breath, edema, dizziness, cramps
Monitoring: BUN/SrCr, LFTs **Counseling:** Take with food			
COX-2 Selective			
MOA: Inhibition of cyclooxygenase resulting in decreased prostaglandins (PG)			
diclofenac tap, cap, gel, patch, topical, solu, inj	VOLTAREN ZORVOLEX	Oral: 50-75 mg BID Zorvolex 18 mg TID	Pruritus, Rash, Site pain
**nabumetone	RELAFEN	1,000-2,000 mg daily	Rash, Pruritus, Tinnitus, edema
celecoxib cap	CELEBREX	200 mg daily or divided	Dyspepsia, Diarrhea
meloxicam tab, cap, susp, oral	MOBIC	7.5-15 mg daily	Abdominal cramps
Contraindication: Sulfonamide allergy, avoid in pregnancy **Monitoring:** BUN/SrCr, LFTs			

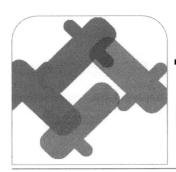

Table 6: Neurological Medications

TABLE 6.1: ANTIPSYCHOTICS

Medication Name		DOSING	ADVERSE REACTION
generic	**BRAND®**		
SECOND GEN ANTIPSYCHOTICS			
aripiprazole inj, ODT, solu, susp	ABILIFY ARISTADA	10-30 MG PO QAM	Tardive Dyskinesia, Anxiety, insomnia
MOA: D2 and 5H2A agonist, 5HT1A partial agonist			
lurasidone	LATUDA	40-160 mg daily	Neuroleptic Malignant Syndrome, Tardive Dyskinesia
MOA: antagonism of dopamine D2 and Serotonin 5HT2 Receptors			
olanzapine	ZYPREXA ZYPREXA ZYDIS ODT	10-20 MG qHS	Agitation, Insomnia, Somnolence, Weight gain, Increase in lipids and glucose,
MOA antagonism of D2 and 5HT Receptors, Inhibitor of Muscarinic/Histamine/Adrenergic alpha-1 Receptors **Monitor: QT, Lipids, Glucose**			
quetiapine	SEROQUEL SEROQUEL XR	400-800 mg daily XR qHS light meal	Dry mouth, Hypotension, Somnolence, Orthostasis, Weight gain,lipid increase
MOA: 5HT1, 5HT2, D2, H1, Adrenergic alpha 1 & 2 Receptors **Monitor:** Metabolic effects			
risperidone	RISPERDAL RISPERDAL ODT	4-16 mg daily	Extrapyramidal symptoms, tachycardia, priapism, weight gain, missed periods
MOA: antagonism of D2 and 5HT2 receptors **Monitoring:** metabolic effects, weight gain			
**ziprasidone	GEODON	40-160 mg **Take with food**	Drowsiness, Heart arrhythmias, dizziness > 8mg increase EPS
MOA: antagonism of D2 and 5HT2 Receptors **Monitoring:** QT, prolactin,			
TRICYCLICS (TCA)			
amitriptyline	ELAVIL	100-300 mg daily qHS	Dry mouth, Blurry vision, Drowsiness, Tachycardia
doxepin	SINEQUAN	100-300 mg daily	
**imipramine	TOFRANIL	100-300 mg daily	
Inhibits reuptake of NE and 5HT at presynaptic nerve terminals			
mirtazapine	REMERON	15 to 45 mg daily	Increased appetite, Weight gain, Dry mouth, Tachycardia
Antagonist of serotonin 5HT2/5HT3 receptors, also inhibitor of H1 and inhibitor of adrenergic alpha-1 muscarinic receptor			
nortriptyline	PAMELOR	25 mg TID-QD	Dry Mouth, Blurry vision, Drowsiness, Tachycardia
Inhibit reuptake of NE and 5HT at presynaptic nerve terminal			

TABLE 6.2: ANTIANXIETY

Medication Name		DOSING	ADVERSE REACTION
generic	BRAND®		

SECOND GEN ANTIPSYCHOTICS

Inhibit reuptake of NE and serotonin at presynaptic nerve terminals.

desvenlafaxine	PRISTIQ KHEDEZLA	50 mg daily	Dry mouth, Constipation, Drowsiness, Tachycardia
duloxetine	CYMBALTA	Initial 30 mg daily	
venlafaxine	EFFEXOR EFFEXOR XR	75-375 mg daily IR 75-225 mg daily ER	

Black Box: Increased suicidal thinking and behavior in children.

SELECTIVE SEROTONIN REUPTAKE INHIBITORS (SSRI)

Inhibits reuptake of 5HT and partial agonist of serotonergic (5-HT) receptors

citalopram	CELEXA	20-40 mg daily	Dry mouth, Constipation, Dizziness, Impotence, Tremor
escitalopram	LEXAPRO	10-40 mg daily	
fluoxetine	PROZAC, SARAFEM	10=60mg daily max 80 mg	
paroxetine	PAXIL, PEXEVA	10-60 mg daily max 75 mg daily	
sertraline	ZOLOFT	50-200 mg daily	

SELECTIVE SEROTONIN REUPTAKE INHIBITORS (SSRIs) AND 5-HT1A PARTIAL AGONIST

vilazodone	VIIBRYD	10 mg x 7 days, then 20 mg daily: **take with food**	Insomnia, decrease libido (less sexual SEs) N/V/D

Contraindication: Seizures, Avoid in patients with linezolid
Boxed: suicidal thinking

TABLE 6.3: BIPOLAR, ADHD AGENTS

Medication Name		DOSING	ADVERSE REACTION
generic	BRAND®		
DOPAMINE AGONIST			
bupropion	WELLBUTRIN, ZYBAN	300-450 mg daily Zyban for smoking cessation 150mg daily	Dry mouth, insomnia, tremors/ seizures, hypertension, sexual disfunction
	MOA: dopamine and NE inhibitor **Boxed:** suicidal behavior　**Contraindication:** Seizure		
CNS AGENT FOR ADHD			
amphetamine and dextroamphetamine salts	ADDERALL ADDERALL XR MYDAYIS	5mg qAM or BID Max 60 mg daily	Dry mouth Restlessness Insomnia Loss of appetite Insomnia Anxiety
	MOA: stimulation on adrenergic receptors, releasing NE **Boxed:** Misuse death, CV issues		
atomoxetine	STRATTERA	40 mg -100 mg daily	
	MOA: inhibition of pre-synaptic NE transporter **Boxed:** suicidal ideation, **CI:** glaucoma **Monitor:** HR, ECG, BP, weight		
**dexmethyl phenidate	FOCALIN	IR: 2.5—20 mg daily ER: 10 -50 mg dialy	
	MOA: central nervous system stimulant)		
lisdexamfetamine	VYVANSE	30 mg to 70 mg qAM	
	MOA: CNS stimulation on adrenergic receptors, releasing NE		
lithium carbonate		300 to 900 mg daily	Diarrhea Drowsiness Vomiting Blurry vision Tinnitus
	MOA: antagonism of NE/Dopamine from nerve terminals, increasing reuptake and inactivation of catecholamine **Monitoring:** 0.5 – 1.2 mEq/L		
methylphenidate tab, chew, oral, patch	RITALIN, METHYLIN METAC	5 mg bid before breakfast 60 mg daily max	Nervousness Insomnia Palpitations
	MOA: Activates the brain stem arousal system and cortex		

TABLE 6.4: PARKINSON'S, ALZHEIMER'S SEEP, MIGRAINE DISORDERS AGENTS

Medication Name		DOSING	ADVERSE REACTION
generic	BRAND®		
PARKINSON'S AGENT			
carbidopa/ levodopa	SINEMET RYTARY ER DUOPE SUSP	IR: 25/100 mg PO TID CR: 50/200 BID	Dystonia, Involuntary movements, N/D, dry mouth, Dementia
	MOA: Carbidopa- inhibits Dopa-Decarboxylase, (increase Levodopa levels); Levodopa converts to dopamine **Contraindication:** MAO inhibitors		
haloperidol IV, tab	HALOPERIDOL	0.5 – 5mg BID, TID	Dystonia, Extrapyramidal reaction, abdominal pain, Hyperkinesia,
	MOA: Postsynaptic D2 receptors in the brain. **Boxed**: Risk of death elderly		
ropinirole	REQUIP REQUIP XL	IR: start with 0.25 mg TID	Somnolence, Syncope, Dizziness
	MOA: D2 and D3 dopamine receptor agonist		
ALZHEIMER'S AGENTS			
MOA: NMDA inhibitor (N-methyl-D-aspartate) which inhibit glutamate form binding to NMDA receptors.			
memantine	NAMENDA NAMENDA XR	IR: 5-10 mg BID ER: 7-28 mg **CrCL < 30:** 5 mg BID **XR**	Dizziness, headache, hallucination
SLEEP AGENTS			
MOA: Inhibits neurotransmitter action of GABA **Counseling:** next-day impairment with < 8 hours of sleep, habit forming, depression, caution with 3A4 inhibitors (azoles, -avir)			
eszopiclone	LUNESTA	1-3 mg qHS **No renal adjustment**	Drowsiness, unpleasant taste dyspepsia, dizziness
zolpidem tab, oral spray, SL	AMBIEN	5-10 mg qHS **No renal adjustment**	Drowsiness, Dry mouth, lethargy, depression
MIGRAINE AGENTS (TRIPTANS)			
MOA: Selective agonist for serotonin ($5\text{-}HT_{1B}$ $5\text{-}HT_{1D}$) in cranial arteries; causes vasoconstriction and reduces migraine.			
rizatriptan	MAXALT	5-10 mg daily repeat after 2 hours max 30 mg/24 hours	Dizziness Drowsiness Nausea

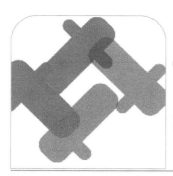

Table 7: Ophthalmic and OTIC Disorders

TABLE 7.1: GLAUCOMA AGENTS

Medication Name			
generic	BRAND®	DOSING	ADVERSE REACTION
BETA-BLOCKERS			
timolol maleate	TIMOPTIC TIMOLOL GFS	1 drop daily or BID shake well first time	Eye irritation, Burning, Signs of systemic absorption, Blurry vision, Stinging, Itching
MOA: Nonselective beta-adrenergic receptor blocker (reduces humor formation and increase outflow) glaucoma agent			
olopatadine	PATANOL, PATADAY		Blurry vision, Burning, Stinging
MOA: Inhibitor of the release of histamine from mast cell (H1 agonist) for eye allergy			
ALPHA 2 AGONIST			
MOA: An alpha-2 adrenergic agonist (reduce production increase outflow) glaucoma agent			
brimonidine	ALPHAGAN	1 drop TID	Allergic conjunctivitis, Eye pruritus, Burning, Sensation
CARBONIC ANHYDRASE INHIBITOR with BETA BLOCKERS			
MOA: Inhibitor of human carbonic anhydrase 2 for glaucoma			
dorzolamide / timolol	COSOPT	**1 DROP BID**	Taste perversion, Burning, Blurry vision
PROSTAGLANDINS			
Synthetic prostaglandin F analogue stimulates prostanoid receptors (increase outflow). glaucoma agent			
bimatoprost **travoprost**	LUMIGAN TRAVATAN	1 Drop qHS	Ocular hyperemia, Blurry vision, Decreased visual acuity
latanoprost	XALATAN	1 DROP qHS Remove contact lenses	Blurry vision, Burning, Stinging eyelashes growth/ thickening Darkening of the iris
MOA: Prostanoid receptor agonist (increase outflow); glaucoma agent			

COUNSELING: Shake eye drop bottle well, wait a few minutes, apply to eyelids. If there are 2 drops wait 3-4 minutes. Some eye drops cause eyelash growth and darkening of eyelashes (prostaglandins) Best to avoid Timolol in patients with **asthma, COPD, and cardiac issues.**

TABLE 7.2: ANTIBIOTICS (OPHTHALMIC)

Medication Name		DOSING	ADVERSE REACTION
generic	BRAND®		
ANTIBIOTICS			
ofloxacin	OCUFLOX	1-2 q2-4h for 2 days 1-2 QID for 5 days	Blurry vision Eye problems
MOA: DNA/RNA inhibitor by interfering with DNA gyrase			
trimethoprim / polymyxin B sulfate	POLYTRIM	1 drop q3h for 7-10 days	Burning Stinging Redness
MOA: Polymyxin B- Disrupts bacterial cell wall Trimethoprim decreases folic acid synthesis			
tobramycin/ dexamethasone	TOBRADEX	1-2 drops q4-6h	Itching, Swelling, Conjunctival erythema
MOA: An Aminoglycosides which binds to 30S and 50S ribosomal units			
neomycin/ polymyxin/ hydrocortisone	CORTISPORIN OTIC	1-2 drops q2-4 for less than 10days	Local irritation Itching Burning
MOA: Neomycin- inhibits the 30S ribosomal unit			
cyclosporin	RESTASIS	1 drop in each eye BID	Burning, Eye pain, Blurry vision
MOA: Unknown (immunomodulation) for dry eys			
naphazoline/ pheniramine	NAPHCON-A VISINE ADV	1-2 drops QID	Mydriasis
MOA: Stimulates alpha-adrenergic receptors in the arterioles of the conjunctiva to produce vaso-constriction.			
ANTIVERTIGO AGENT			
meclizine	ANTIVERT	25 – 100 mg daily or BID	Drowsiness Dry mouth
MOA: Histamine (H1) receptor blocker			

TABLE 7.4: ANTIALLERGENS

Medication Name			
generic	BRAND®	DOSING	ADVERSE REACTION
**cypro-heptadine	PERIACTIN	weight based dosing	Drowsiness, Dry mouth, Blurry vision
	MOA: Inhibitor of H_1 receptor and Serotonin (5-HT) receptor		
Benzonatate	TESSALON PERLES ZONATUSS	100-200 mg daily	Drowsiness, Nasal congestion, Burning eyes
	MOA: Anesthetizes stretch receptors, dampening their activity and reducing cough reflex		
hydroxyzine hydrochloride	ATARAX	10 mg/ 4 mL	Drowsiness, Dry mouth
	MOA: Antagonizes H1 receptors (CNS)		
hydroxyzine pamoate	VISTARIL	25-50 mg daily	Drowsiness, Dry mouth
	MOA: Antagonizes H1 receptors (peripheral tissues)		
diphen-hydramine cap, tab, chew, elixir, strip, syrup, susp, inj, cream, gel,	BENADRYL	25-50 mg q4-6h max 300 mg/day	Somnolence, cognitive impairment, anticholinergic effects (dry mouth, vision)
	MOA: Antagonizes H1 receptors		
2nd GEN ANTIHISTAMINES (H_1) Antagonize H1 receptors			
loratadine tab, cap, chew, solu, ODT	CLARITIN Claritin-D 24h	5-10 mg daily	Somnolence
azelastine	ASTELIN, ASTEPRO	1-2 spray per nostril BID	Bitter taste, Drowsiness, Dry mouth, Nasal burning
cetirizine	ZYRTEC ZYRTEC-D	5-10 mg daily (max 5 mg)	Somnolence, occasionally
levocetirizine	XYZAL	5 mg qHS	Dry mouth, Somnolence, Nasopharyngitis

TABLE 7.5: ANTIALLERGENS (CONT..)

Medication Name			
generic	BRAND®	DOSING	ADVERSE REACTION
ANALGESICS WITH ANTIPYRETICS			
promethazine/ codeine	PHENEGRAN /CODEINE	6.25mg/10mg per 5 mL every 4 to 6 hours, PRN	Drowsiness Hypogonadism
**hydrocodone/ chlorpheniramine	TUSSIONEX	10 mg/ 8mg BID	Decreased mental alertness Hypotension, hypersensitivity
		Boxed: respiratory depression including fatalities especially in children	
ANTITUSSIVE			
promethazine/ dextromethorphan	PHENEGRAN -DM	15MG/6.25 mg 5 mL q4-6h PRN (max 30)	Drowsiness, Constipation
EXPECTORANTS			
MOA: Guaifenesin- thinning bronchial secretion, lubrication, facilitating removal. Codeine- depresses the cough reflex center in the medulla oblongata.			
codeine/ guaifenesin	ROBAFEN AC VITUSSIN AC	100 mg / 10 mg per 5 mL 10 mL PO q4h PRN 60 mL per day	Drowsiness, constipation

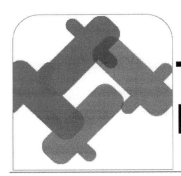

Table 8: Respiratory Disorder Medications

TABLE 8.1 :ANTIASTHMATICS

Medication Name		DOSING	ADVERSE REACTION
generic	BRAND®		
ICS (INHALED CORTICOSTEROIDS)			
MOA: Adrenocorticoids form steroid-receptor complex. Help in m-RNA synthesis (anti-inflammatory) actions **Contraindication:** First line agent for status asthmaticus or acute exacerbation **Duration: 5 to 7 days** **Monitor:** Asthma response (SABA)			
beclomethasone 40,80 mg/INH	QVAR	MD: 1-4 INH BID	Pharyngitis Nasa Congestion
budesonide 90, 180 mcg/INH	PULMICORT	DPI: 1-4 INH BID	URTI, Oral candidiasis
fluticasone HFA 110, 220 mcg/INH Elipta: 100, 200 mcg/INH	FLOVENT	MDI: 2 INH BID DPI: 1-2 IINH daily	Dysphonia (difficulty speaking) Oral candidiasis (thrush) Cough, Headache, URTIs
SYSTEMIC STEROIDS			
methyl prednisolone oral	SOLU-MEDROL	IV: LD 1mg/kg 30 minutes, taper dose	
prednisolone oral	ORAPED	Oral: 5 to 60 mg daily	Blurry vision GI upset
prednisone oral	DELTASONE	30 mg daily in divided dose	Fluid/electrolyte issues Local burning or Itching
clobetasol propionate topical	TEMOVATE	Topical for 2 weeks	Hyperglycemia Fluid retention Weight gain
hydrocortisone topical	ANUSOL-HC PROCTOSOL-HC	Asthma??: 200 mg divided	
triamcinolone topical	KENALOG	Allergies: 40 to 80 mg daily	
LEUKOTRIENE INHIBITORS			
montelukast	SINGULAIR	5-10 mg qHS	Headache, influenza, abdominal pain; neuropsychiatric events
	Inhibits physiologic actions of LTD4		
PHOSPHODIESTERASE PDE III INHIBITORS			
**theophylline	THEO-24	ER: 300-600 mg daily	Tachycardia, N/V, Seizures, Hypokalemia
	MOA: bronchodilation by suppression process		

TABLE 8.2: COPD AGENTS

Medication Name		DOSING	ADVERSE REACTION
generic	BRAND®		
LAAC (LONG-ACTING ANTICHOLINERGICS)			
MOA: Antagonist of acetylcholine at M3 and M1 receptors with cholinergic effects of bronchoconstriction and mucus secretion			
tiotropium bromide 18 mcg daily	SPIRIVA RESPIMAT	DPI: 1 CAP HandiHaler MDI: 2 INH daily	Dry mouth Chest pain, Respiratory infection Tachycardia
**aclidinium 400 mcg BID	TUDORZA	DPI: 1 INH BID	
** umeclidinium	INCRUSE	DPI: 1 INH daily	
SABA (SHORT-ACTING BETA-BLOCKER)			
MOA: Stimulates adenyl cyclase (beta-2-agnoist)			
albuterol sulfate	PROVENTIL PROAIR	MDI: 90 mcg/spray, PRN	Nausea Nervousness Tachycardia

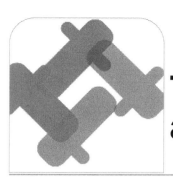

Table 9: Reproductive and Urinary Disorders

TABLE 9.1: AGENTS FOR ERECTILE DYSFUNCTION, OVERACTIVE BLADDER, PROSTATE and GOUT

Medication Name		DOSING	ADVERSE REACTION
generic	BRAND®	DOSING	ADVERSE REACTION
PDE-5 INHIBITORS			
MOA: Increase CGMP causing smooth muscles relaxation allowing inflow of blood to the penis.			
sildenafil citrate	VIAGRA REVATIO	50-100 mg daily **CrCl >65, Renal**	Flushing, Prolonged erection, Headache, Dyspepsia, Blurred vision, Diarrhea, Myalgia
tadalafil	CIALIS	2.5-5 mg daily **CrCl 30-50 mg/min:: 5 mg** PRN **CrCl <30 5 mg PRN, Q72**	
	CONTRAINDICATIONS: NITRATES! **Monitoring:** B <90/50 mmHg, Priapism > 4 hrs		
ANTICHOLINERGIC DRUGS			
MOA: Inhibits Muscarinic action of acetylcholine on smooth muscle (relaxes bladder smooth muscle); a competitive muscarinic receptor antagonist			
oxybutynin tab, topical, gel, patch	DITROPAN	5-30 mg PO daily	Dizziness and Drowsiness (Oxybutynin), Xerostomia (dry mouth), , Agitation, Blurry vision, Urinary retention,
solifenacin succinate	VESICARE	5—10 mg PO daily	
tolterodine **tolterodine ER**	DETROL DETROL LA	1-2 mg BID 2-4 mg daily	
****phenazopyridine**	PYRIDIUM	Two (190 mg) TID	
	Counseling: Take with food.		
ANTIGOUT			
MOA: Inhibition of the migration of granulocytes into the inflamed area.			
colchicine	CLOCRYS	Two 0.6 mg tab, and 0.6 mg in 1 hour **CrCl < 30 mL/ min**	Vomiting, Myelosuppression Diarrhea, Myopathy Nausea
	Monitoring: CBC, LFTs, renal functions **Use:** For actue gout attack with NSAIDs or steroids		
allopurinol	ZYLOPRIM	100-300 mg daily **CrCl<20: max 200 mg**	Rash, Abdominal Pain Diarrhea hypersensitivity, HLA*5801
	MOA: Inhibits Xanthine Oxidase **Monitoring:** CBC, LFTs, renal function **Level:** titrate to a target level of < 6 mg/dL uric acid.		

TABLE 9.2: MENOPAUSE, ANTINEOPLASTIC

Medication Name			
generic	BRAND®	DOSING	ADVERSE REACTION
			ANTINEOPLASTIC
anastrozole	ARIMIDEX	1 mg daily	Vasodilation Asthenia, Localized pain Decreases in bone mineral density and increases in serum cholesterol
***letrozole*	*FEMARA*	2.5 mg once daily	
MOA: Selective non-steroidal competitive aromatase inhibitor *(binds to heme CYP450)*			
methotrexate	METHOTREXATE	5 - 30 mg daily-weekly	Weak Immune Response, Rash, Nephrotoxicity, Hepatotoxicity, Cough
MOA: Inhibits Dihydrofolic acid Reductase, (interferes with DNA synthesis, repair, cellular replications) **may require:** Leucovorin			
azathioprine	IMURAN	50 mg q12h	
MOA: Azathioprine is cleaved to 6-*MP*, which in turn, is converted to additional metabolites that inhibit *de novo* purine synthesis.			
tamoxifen	SOLTAMOX	20 mg daily	DVT/PE, hot flashes, flushing, edema, weight gain, hypertension, mod changes
MOA: Selective Estrogen Receptor Modulators (SERM)			

Made in the USA
Monee, IL
03 October 2023

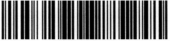